On the Other Side
of the Bed Pan

ON THE OTHER SIDE OF THE BED PAN

Pat Martin LPN
(Retired)

To order additional copies of this book, contact:
Xlibris Corporation
1-888-795-4274
www.Xlibris.com
Orders@Xlibris.com
54269

CONTENTS

DEDICATION

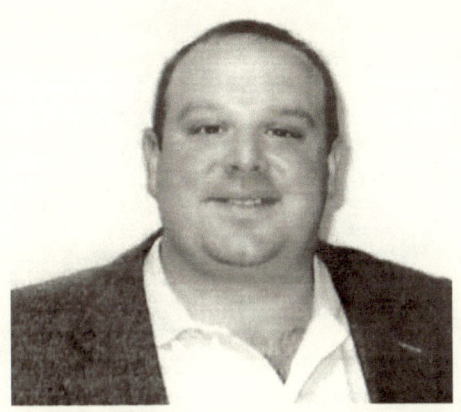

Doctor Richard Tallarico, my surgeon and friend.

You stood by me even when I was off the wall and was swearing and telling stupid stories. You would say your right Pat and leave and come back the next day and ask if I had been dreaming and I would say "no, I think I was hallucinating." You told me before the surgery everything that was going to happen or may happen. I sat there and said to my self that is not going to happen to me. In a week I will be trucking down the hill, because I was a health professional and was one up on most people. Boy did I ever have to eat crow, after a week I was just getting out of ICU. You have given me a new lease on life. I am pain free, and able to sleep in a bed and walk down the street which I was not able to do in the past two years. Even though you made me drink that terrible Ensure three times a day for four weeks, I was a much nicer person. I brought you Girl Scout cookies. I will hold you to that drink you said we would have when this is over. After three surgeries and two infections and lots of swearing on my part I can finally see the light at the end of the tunnel, and you are still there for me and my family. Thank you from the bottom of my heart. You kept telling me not to get depressed. I think you realized that I'm not one to get depressed but I get mad and really pissed off when things don't go the way I expected them to.

Prelude

They say Doctors and Nurses make the worst patients. I agree one hundred percent. I was always the giver and never the receiver, always in control of everything. This is why I decided on the name. *ON THE OTHER SIDE OF THE BED PAN*. I had to depend on someone to wash and feed me and wipe my ass. I had no control over my bodily functions. It was the worst experience of my life, perhaps my story will be a help to some other patient.

CHAPTER 1

Background

Where do I start? I guess by telling you a little about myself. I am a sixty seven year old retired LPN and was in good health until an old back injury from the seventies and eighties reoccured and became a big problem after twenty years. It was a change that came on slowly until I could no longer walk one block without pain. Before this I walked eighteen holes on the golf course and played in five leagues without a problem, and cared for my family and my home. I have my husband George of forty five years, one son George Jr., three daughters Patty, Debbie and Kim, nine grandchildren and Sandy our 10 year old dog.

First I had to have bilateral knee replacement and then my back started to give me problems. I would take anti-inflamatories and pain meds, prescribed by my family physician and at first they would help. Then I couldn't sleep through the night with the pains in my right hip and back. I scheduled an appointment with my Orthopedic Physician Doctor Dave but by the time I got in to see him the pain had gone from my right hip and was in my left hip and down the front of both legs. I asked Doctor Dave if I should see an Arthritis doctor because I thought it was my back not my hip. He sent me to Dr. Shell whom in turn had me get a Bone Scan and an MRI. Dr. Shell also had me have a nerve conductor test and then he sat down with me and said I had to see Doctor Bob the spinal surgeon. Then the fun began.

February 2007 I got in to see doctor Bob. In the mean time I was sleeping in my recliner at night. I was unable to walk a block or do house work and it was a chore to do the shopping. I was in constant pain. This went on until my surgery in January of 2008. Doctor Bob said I needed to have ten discs of my spine operated on and involves a fusion and rods and screws.

I got three separate opinions and everyone said the same that if I did not have surgery I would end up in a wheel chair within a couple years. I had to have a bone density and my spinal bones came back good to put the screws into. I had Stenosis and Scoliosis

Every time I went to see Doctor Bob he kept saying the catholic hospital would not buy him the machine he needed for my surgery. I was to have the surgery in July of 2007. When he was denied again, Doctor Bob said he was sending me to a doctor he would use for himself. That is how I met Dr. T at the teaching hospital. The fun was just beginning.

CHAPTER 2

Encounter

October 9th 2007 was the big day. I was upset when I walked into Doctor T office. I was in pain and had been for so long, I was not a happy camper. I believe it was the meeting of the Irishman and the Italian. He never told me until long after my surgery that he knew I was pissed off because he would not do surgery until he completed all his own test and not use Dr. Bob's that I brought with me. Also I was to quit smoking for six weeks prior to my surgery. He asked me to try and lose twenty pounds. I told him that he had a better chance to see God then me quitting smoking and also losing weight. I would probably gain weight.

X-rays, MRI, Bone Scan and standing back x-Rays where scheduled along with me seeing a Hematologist because of my blood disorder (Thala Simia Minor) and my next appointment was made. I went right out in Doctor T's, parking lot and smoked two cigarettes. Didn't know that did you Doc? By the time I got home my poor husband must have thought his wife had flipped out. I was just ranting and raving. I hurt so bad that I would have done anything to get relief. So I settled down and it took two weeks for me to quite smoking. The hardest place was the Legion Post where quite a few smokers come in. In December I saw Doctor T again, by then I had completed all the test and x-rays that had to be done and had gone to the blood doctor and was cleared in that department. Things were starting to come together. By the second visit Doctor T and I were hitting it off better and I realized every thing he ordered was for my own good. He even had me go to Aquatics Therapy which felt great while in the water. I did say no when he wanted to give me a Nerve block in my back. I won out on that one. I had many of those in late 1979 and 1982. Doctor T said that was in the dark ages but I said no—no—no. So it stayed no.

No I did not lose twenty pounds but I did lose three, better than gaining. Sorry doc. I had quite smoking by this time. Cat, the nurse, told me I had to have a nicotine test. By this time I would not have lied to them. The test came back fine.

Doctor T spoke to me again about the surgery and what it entailed. Two days of surgery and time in ICU. Sure like I believed him! I was not going to be like that. I was going to be out of there in a week. One week I was just getting out of ICU. I was a mess. I had to eat crow and admit to the doctor he was right. Lord I hate saying I was wrong. I thought I knew my body but Dr. T knew it better than I. Ouch! I bite my tongue on that one. I had to sign my surgery authorization and an authorization form to resuscitate me as Doctor T said I was not going to die on his watch and I said "I better not because I would come back and haunt him". I was told at this time that I had to stop my anti-inflamitory meds ten days prior to surgery and a couple of my other pills.

By the time I was off the pills one week I was in such pain that I was crawling to the bathroom on my hands and knees. I had to call Nurse Cat and she ordered Hydrocodone. I had told one of my kids that if I had to live with this pain this is not quality of life and I did not care if I died during the surgery. Sorry doc it's a good thing this surgery came out so good because I wouldn't have wanted to haunt you. You're too nice a guy.

CHAPTER 3

Admission and Surgery

January 28 2008 I awoke and showered at 4:30am. The last shower I had for the next four months. My husband George, daughter Debbie and my self took off for the hospital, my last time to drive for three months. My daughter Patty and granddaughter Kristy met us there. Once I stepped onto the circle there is little that I remember for the next week. I was told that we went to admissions and then from there to the OR holding area and was put in room one. I don't even remember what I wore to the hospital or getting my self undressed or even seeing Doctor T. before the surgery.

My grandson Christopher who works nights in housekeeping was there also and told me some doctor came in and gave me something in my IV. Christopher said within a few seconds I was telling him he should try some of this shit. It was good stuff and legal. He kept saying granny. He said I kept talking about my out laws and in laws, what ever that was.

My family said that the first day of the operation took eight hours. Doctor T spoke to them for quite some time after it was over and said he decompressed the discs and put the screws in. He expected me to go through 2200cc of fluid but I used 4400cc. He said I was taken to ICU and would be there until the second stage of the surgery in a couple days. I was given six units of blood during the surgery and another five units over the next two days because they were trying to get my crit up. My family said the doctors had to do a lot of catching up due to my blood lose.

My daughter Patty took a picture of me the day after the surgery. When I saw it I had so much fluid I looked like a beached whale with a small head. Doctor T you told me I may have to go to ICU. You knew I was going there.

I was told I was bad in ICU. I kept trying to pull my lines out and needed to be restrained, when my hands were tied then I used my legs like I was peddling a bike. I remember none of this. I do know I had a dream before my admission that I woke up with the tube down my throat and guess what? It did happen and I thought I was going to choke to death. I remember seeing Patty and Debbie standing on each side of the bed and Patty saying mom is trying to say something. I was trying to say I can't breath and here they are standing there trying to figure out what I wanted and I was going to die before they figured it out. So I thought I will spell it in the air with my finger. "I can't breath". Patty said why she is drawing circles. I wanted to smash both their heads together. Finally Debbie said I think she is spelling I can't breath and I nodded yes. Don't worry mom you can breathe around the tube Debbie told me. "You lay here and tell me you can breathe around it". I must have fallen back asleep and when I awoke the tube was out and guess who was standing there, and I think I called him a fu—a—ho—none other than Doctor T. I got thinking about it and said I better apologize, so when he came in again I can just remember him saying (No you didn't do that. But I'm pretty sure I did and my niece Laurie said "yes you did". So again, I'm sorry doc. I was told that I called a lot of people a lot of different names and gave them my special blessing and it involved my middle finger. It's probably a good thing that they give you meds to make you forget. Sometime around now I was measured for my turtle shell. That's what I called it. I don't remember only that it arrived in the unit and I was to wear it at some point.

Laurie, what was the tassels you wanted to put on the front of my lovely shell (brace) that was made for me? Just remember pay back is a bitch. Some day yours will come.

All I remember are flashes of things and being very pissed off. But I can't remember why. Debbie said it may have been when the nurses were turning me and doing things to me. They felt bad because they knew I was hurting. I do not remember any of this. You are given medication to make you not remember what is happening.

CHAPTER 4

Second Stage of Surgery

January 31st, I remember very little of the last two days. I know they moved me to the Orthopedic Floor for a couple hours. They needed the bed in ICU for incoming emergency. I was told later that they put a vena cava filter in me so I would not get blood clots. This will remain in me for life. George said they took me from the room to do this procedure under fluoroscopic. I can just remember the orthopedic floor and at this time I hated it. I thought some woman sat up all night on a couch, George said it was in a chair she was sitting, I thought that I was in a closet. Man, I was so confused. I never remember going to surgery again. This was when the rods were put in and everything was connected.

George said I went through another four units of blood and 2200cc of fluids and after eight hours of surgery I was put back in ICU for another couple of days. Man that is another part of my life that is gone, kaput or something. I was told that I did guilt trips on my kids. I told them if they left me alone I would die. They kept saying we have to go home it's 11pm and we have to get the kids on the bus for school in the morning. You know if I was myself I would never do anything like that.

Doctor T told me that he was present when they were waking me up and the tube was removed, the nurse said, "Pat your surgery is over" and the first thing I said was "no shit". It's weird how I remember none of this.

I remember Kim coming up but only the day they were moving me to the Orthopedic floor again and I know I was yelling I didn't want to go there. Everyone said George was there every day sitting by my bed I only remember grabbing for his hand now and then. My family told me that doctor T. would come in and speak to them but I knew nothing about it. I was in la-la land. Tomorrow I get transferred to Ortho.

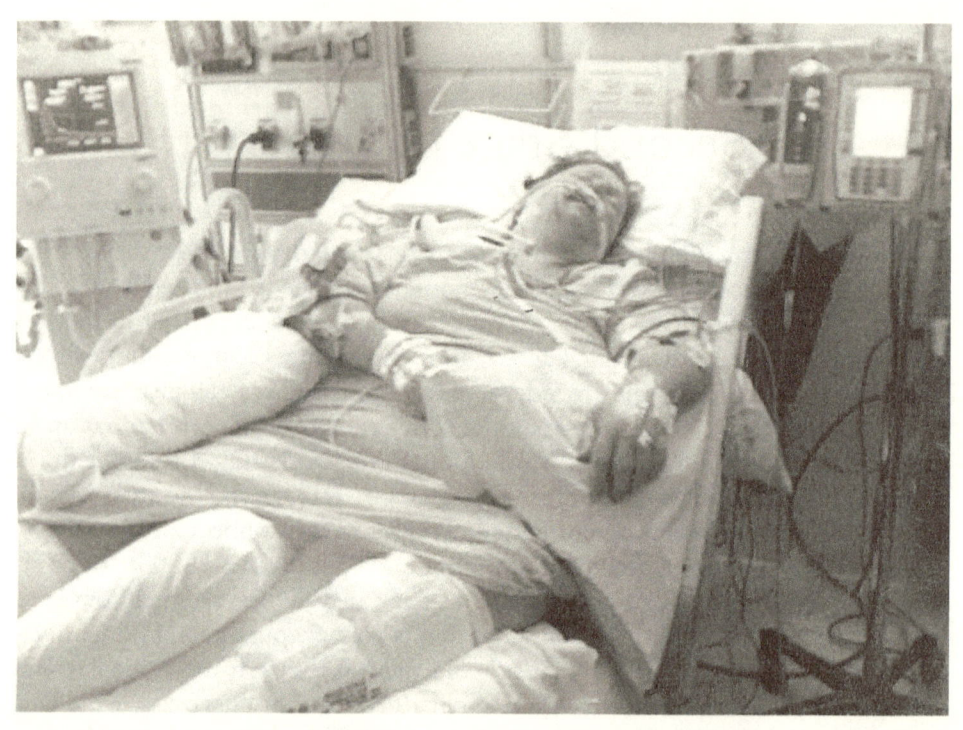

Pat—second day in ICU—(did not know myself.)

CHAPTER 5

Orthopedic Floor

I do not remember leaving ICU and I was quite confused the first few days on my new floor. I think the morphine was doing a number on me. I can remember doctor T coming to my room and talking to me but I only remember the conversation about pumping my feet like pressing on the gas pedal and the break in a car and to keep doing it until my shins hurt. This was to prevent me from getting blood clots. I remember telling him that my shins never hurt because I keep falling asleep.

Around this time the priest from my parish came to visit me. It was about 7:30am. I have no idea what we talked about but I do know I only had my night shirt on and no covers. I pray I was some what decent. When I got home he came to my house and said, "we had a nice conversation in the hospital". I can just imagine what I talked about, I probably gave him a blessing or two.

Every time I got up I had to have that turtle shell put on before getting out of bed. It was way too big as I was measured when I was full of fluid in ICU. So the fitter came back and took it back to the shop with him. The brace was returned in a couple hours. I was told I was to learn to put it on before I got out of bed. You got to be kidding. There is no way I will ever be able to get into this thing while I'm in bed. It takes two from the floor to put it on while I'm in bed. After they got me up, then the adjusting began even Doctor T tried to adjust the darn thing. The doctor asked me if I thought the brace might be making the opening in my incision worse. Don't ask me I have no idea. I'm so confused I'm not sure what end is up.

I had no pain, just muscle spasms and I kept telling Doctor T that I was free of pain. He said don't tell people I don't give pain because I do. All I know is I had no pain.

I hate this floor already and I've only been here a day and I would love to leave. Everyone is running around and slamming doors. It is so noisy and very warm. They got me a fan and it did help some.

I know I went for x rays late in the evening. I was left down there by myself and then the tech wanted me to stand by myself. He gave me an IV pole to hang on to and it had wheels. Once I stood and locked my knees I did all right, but to get to my feet was another chore. Someone should be with you and not be left alone down there. I was so afraid to stand up alone and the tech was not going to help.

Ever since I woke from surgery I have had no feeling from my waist to my toes, but this slowly is coming back. I would get all these pins and needles. After about three weeks all the feeling came back in my left leg and foot. The right leg and hip is still numb from just above the knee up my thigh and about a two inch band across the top edge of the cheeks of my rear. I swear Doctor T put a self adjusting screw in my right hip and the more I move the more it tightens. Sounds crazy but that is how it feels to me. This numbness and pressure still continues to this day July 1st, 2008.

At this point I was so confused. My family would ask me a question and I thought I was answering them right off. They said maybe ten minutes later I would reply. Patty said she asked Dr. T what was wrong with me. He told her it was all the medication I had taken. He told her some people swear up and down that he brings licorice to them at midnight. I didn't have that problem but I did take an un-scheduled walk out of bed one night and fell on the floor.

This is one story I want to forget. I remember nothing of getting out of bed. I thought I heard a siren. They had taken the catheter out of me and had twice straight catherized me. I had to go to bathroom. I guess I climbed out of bed over the side rail and the first recollection I had was standing in the middle of the floor without my brace or walker and I was falling. I was afraid of dislodging the screws so I went to my knees. I then peed on the floor. If I could have gotten myself back into the bed and never told anyone what I did, it would have been fine with me.

I tried calling my room mate to ring her bell. She was sleeping. So I crawled to the bed on my hands and knees and started to pull the linen off the bed and pulled the call bell out of the wall which in turn made the light outside my door come on. Two male nurses came in the room talking to each other and then said, "where is she," "I'm down here on the floor", was my reply, "watch where you are stepping". I was so embarrassed. So many reports had to be made out and my doctor had to be called.

Guess who was in my room about 5:30am? Your one hundred percent right Doctor T. First thing he asked "was I confused?". No, I was sleeping and woke up standing in the room and starting to fall. He asked if I should have my knees x rayed. I said, "absolutely not, lets just forget the whole thing". I felt like some doddering old fool. Of course they gave me the lovely bracelet that people who fall have to wear at all times and need someone with you when out of bed.

I think I told Doctor T at some point he had two heads with horns. At least I think I remember that, maybe I was dreaming. Man I was a fruit cake.

About this time I was having a big problem being able to get on the commode without wetting myself as I had no muscles to hold my urine when they stood me up to get on the commode and I would start peeing right off. I also had a very hard time having a bowel movement. I swore I would never be like this and worry about these bodily functions that all the old people worried about when I took care of them. I wanted to be remembered as the dirty minded old lady who always talked about sex. Wrong again I was either wetting or pooping myself or giving the bird or swearing. Great this is what I wanted to be remembered for. Doctor T this was one subject you did not discuss with me, bowel and bladder control.

I started going down to physical therapy for ambulation with a walker. I was so weak. I could not get out of bed without help. I was unable to lift my left leg off the bed I thought I had a stroke and was afraid to say anything to any one.

I also had a problem with my incision. Some of it had opened up due to my stomach and the swelling I had. Doctor T. said he was going to have a plastic surgeon look at the wound and an infection control doctor and get their opinion. Of course they don't tell me a thing because I'm not their patient. Well thank you very much. They said, "ask Doctor T, he is your doctor".

Just about this time the interviewer from the Rehab floor came to speak to me about my transfer to their unit. That was fine with me. It was one more step closer to going home. I would do anything to get off this floor. After falling no one wanted to get me up. Doctor T wanted me out of bed and moving so as to prevent blood clots. The staff kept putting me off. On Saturday night I told the staff you better get me up because they were going to have one mad doctor if I was still in bed in the morning when he made his rounds. So I finely talked the staff into getting me up. I told them if I put the effort into getting out of bed you can put the effort into helping me up. So between midnight and 6am in the morning I got up five times and put out seven hundred to one thousand cc each time I got up. They had to use some kind of bumper machine with a lift to get me out of bed. Dr. T laughed when he came in that morning and seen how often I had got out of bed. I told him what my conversation was with the staff.

About the same day nurse aide Lou had me for a patient, Lou washed my hair the first in a week or more. Did that ever feel great. She was working with nurse pony tail. The aide did all five of their patients that they had together. She washed and bathed all five patients herself. I told nurse pony tail how lazy she or he was. The only thing that person did all day was pass meds to five patient and stayed in the med room and shut off their Vercvo phone.

The aide washed my hair and she assisted me out of bed and once I stood up and locked my knees I could stand. I looked out the window and said my daughter Patty works on the rock right next to where the tractor trailer is tipped over. That never happened, I kept seeing spiders flying around and I was telling Lou to kill them. When she helped me back into bed I said I can't believe some one would draw that on the wall under the television. She said, "What is that?" why the two big boobs with tits on the end. It was the cords from the televisions going to the outlets. Boy was I crazy or what. I'm surprised a straight jacket was not ordered for me. Everyone must have had fun reading my chart. All the crazy stuff I talked about that never happened. I told the staff and the doctor to take the morphine pump from me. I refused to use it ever again as it was making me nuts. Once it was discontinued and I started to receive oral medication I was back to my normal, only slightly nutty self.

Tomorrow I will be going to Rehab. Thank god I'm leaving here. Maybe it's just me being so mixed up, but this is not a floor I want to stay on, it is so confusing here or I am just confused. One more step closer to going home or should I say one more rotation of the wheel chair as I'm not walking yet.

CHAPTER 6

Rehab Floor

George came up and I was taken to rehab in a wheel chair, the next step on the road to recovery. I still had lots of fluid in me. I was weight upon my arrival to rehab and still had over fifty pounds to lose. I was introduced to so many people and I was having problems with names I was so forgetful. I was given a shower schedule but of course because of my open incision I was unable to shower on my days Tuesday and Thursday. All I could do was sponge bathe.

I was given a room by myself and I was alone most of the four weeks. I enjoyed that because I am a poor sleeper and was up most of the nights, So I was not disturbing anyone, even now that I'm home I still get up a couple nights a week around 4:00 or 5:00 am.

This sounds crazy but the night staff and I would take bets as to how much urine I put out every two hours. Guess who would win, yours truly. It was just something to do to pass the time. We would laugh.

I was signed off to the rehab doctor upon admission Doctor Way. My own physician Doctor T came every day to see me and check my wound. I think at this point he was seeing more of me then he saw his family. He would sit and talk to me and tell me about his family. He is a very caring person.

I was in rehab only one day when I had a big problem. Doctor T said if they wanted to change my dressing one hundred times a day they could but he did not want them to touch the wound. Well guess what, one Resident tried to squeeze the open incision and I told him to stop. It was written up that I was un—cooperative also they wanted to wash the site with saline. So when Dr. T came in the next day with his entourage, which included the supervisor from the floor, I asked him what he said he repeated what we had discussed. Apology was given and accepted.

Some of the staff was upset with me because I could not wipe my behind after a bowel movement. It upset me because I had stitches in the crack of my butt and was afraid if I used the handy tool they gave me I would get stool into my incision. So I would ask the staff to do it and guess what? They wiped it into the stitches. I could not wipe without the fancy tool I was given, due to my short arms. I'm sure this was discussed because Dr. T even checked it out and had me stand up and he said "You do have short arms". I told him if he had this surgery he would have the same problem as he has short arms.

I was given a schedule for my daily routine. I was to be in Physical Therapy at 8:00 am. So I got up at 5or 5:30am, had the staff put me in the bathroom, give me my clothes, wash cloth and towel and I would wash what I could reach. They would help me get dressed. I had a problem reaching below my knees, so needless to say my lower legs, behind and back I could not reach. I needed someone to wash my hair and help me put on my pants, socks and shoes. I was not going to beg someone to do this for me so I would ask my daughters to help me. They said something to the staff that my mother needs help with her hygiene.

At this point I said something to Doctor T. that rehab was great for getting you going but hygiene meant a lot to me and no one was washing my hair or my stockings and my feet. My kids were told that I refused hygiene. Patty said my mother gets up every day at home at 6:00am showers and washes her hair. I don't believe she would refuse because she is very up set over this and I want something done. Needless to say things improved in this department.

Breakfast was at 7:30am, Physical Therapy 8:00-9:00am. Occupational Therapy 9:00-10:00am, Recreational Therapy at 10:00 until 11:00am and then I would stay and have lunch in Recreational therapy. After lunch it was back to Physical Therapy from 1:00 until 2:00 then OT and finished for the day at 3:00 pm. It was a busy day and I usually took a nap when I was through. Fridays was donut day with Ms. Dawn, you could order what ever kind of Danish that you wanted. My favorite was headlights. This was the schedule five days a week.

Weekends were very long and boring unless recreational Therapist Mr. Peter came in and showed movies or played games with us on Sunday. Mass in the chapel was at 10:00am. The second Sunday that I was there we played Wii an interactive video game. This was to help strengthen muscles and coordination. I played golf and played two holes then I slept for two hours. I get so tired, but hate sleeping during the day because then I have problems sleeping at night. I told doctor T on Monday I played golf Sunday and he look at me like I had a brain relapse. I like to tease Doctor T he is so serious I explained about the game wii.

My daughter Debbie has a girlfriend she went to school with twenty odd years ago. Debbie came to see me and I was telling her about the visit I had from her girl friend's mother one night at 2:00am. She flushed my pic line and sat and spoke to me for a couple hours. Debbie said, "mom, it never happened." The friend's mother is over eighty years old and was not a nurse. She was a starving artist. I swear it was so real even to this day I believe she was there.

I had a problem with numbers, putting them in order and also peoples' names. So Recreational Therapist Dawn would sit and play cards with me. The first week or so she could beat me but as my mind improved I would beat her. After a couple weeks I could collate the numbers in the right order. I told Ms. Dawn that if I had to play bingo I was going home. Lord, I hate that game. At first I thought going to rehab was foolish. In my head I thought I was fine physical and mentally. I argued with the kids and George I was not confused and could take care of myself. I think back how dependent I was on everyone.

It takes a long time to accept the things I can do and realize the things I can't do. This is still a big problem for me. I feel I can do everything I always did, and I want to do everything.

George was learning to put the brace on so I can get up. I hate this thing. It is still too big due to me losing more of my excess fluid. I will never be able to put this on in bed by myself. Maybe if they let me up, then I could get it on myself. The day Patty helped her father adjust the thing I thought I was going to never be able to breathe again. Her hands are so strong they both cranked it up on each side I couldn't move. It is still too big. Doctor T said contact the company again. The rep came and took it back. I said make sure you get it right back as I won't be able to get out of bed. He had it back in a couple hours. It's much better It's not loose any more.

About this time Doctor T said "I think the brace is making the open incision worse." So he does not want me wearing it anymore and see what happens. I was just as happy to be without it. I believe the staff was happy also.

It felt good to start being active. George would help me walk and transfer me to the bed or toilet. I would take a short nap every afternoon. Both George and Kim were cleared by Bobbie in Physical therapy so they could walk me and help me to the bathroom and help to get me into bed. At this time I was in wheel chair and could only walk very short distances. I was taking pain meds for the muscle spasms. This would make me very sleepy.

My kids have seen me naked more times during my hospital stay then any time they were growing up. They even had to put my pants on me. They were like the parent and me the child. To have someone do these things for me was very hard for me to accept I was always the giver not the receiver. Even now August 11, 2008 I came home from water therapy without my socks on. I refused to ask someone to put them on. I had a problem with them today.

I did different exercises in PT, walking with help, leg and arm exercises with weights. OT would have me stand for balance and fold clothes, put nuts and bolts together and putting different sticks into holes, or we would play cards and it helped my memory. I guess all the medication is finely leaving my body.

My physical therapist was always kidding with my husband and myself. She would tell me she was meeting George on the side. Boy would he blush. Bobby said how great my new bed that George purchased since I came in here and they were making sure it was going to be good for my back. Bobby, you knew how to cheer someone up. The saying goes something about all work and no play makes someone a dull boy. And it sure was not dull around you. Thanks.

To find someone worse off then me all I had to do was look around. Head injuries, strokes, paralyzed patients. Lord there for the grace of God could be me. When I was first admitted most of the clients could not speak or function. But as the days went by they were doing more for their self. Catheters were being removed and IV's were taken out and the clients were starting to feed themselves, some were even speaking. I guess I should be thankful that I could express my self and say what I wanted. Brother could I ever express myself. I never had any trouble in that department. I think sometimes they wished I would be quiet. Ha Ha.

The first day in rehab I was asked what my goals were in regards to going home. I told the boss lady, Doctor Way, that I was aiming to go home tomorrow. She said, "be realistic about this". I said, "one week and I would go home". In just one week I was back in surgery due to infection of e-coli in my incision. The day Doctor T. had to tell me he was taking me back into surgery I believe he wanted to be anywhere else but in my room. I'm sorry I got so mad. If I could have walked out of there I would have. I knew I would have been taking my problems with me. This was not an option.

You said you may have to give me a wound vac. You already knew that you were going to have to do this. You just did not want to tell me. Again you had the plastic surgeon take a look at the incision and again he said he could tell me nothing. I had to speak to Doctor T. I just love these guys. It's my body.

The morning of February 13th was the day of my surgery. Ms.Dawn came and sat with me in my room. I was NPO and my husband was sick at home and Ms. Dawn knew I was upset about going to surgery again so she spent the morning with me 12:00noon I was taken over to surgery, before I left I was told I could come back to rehab if I promised to go to PT the next morning. All I know I did not want to go back to the orthopedic floor. I would have stood on my head if it meant I was staying on Rehab. At 3:00pm I was taken into surgery. Lord I hate to be put to sleep. I'm so bad when I wake up from surgery. I could hear someone yelling in the recovery room "its fu—cold in here". You guessed it, it was me and I could hear someone say "she's back". Doctor T said it was his resident, Doctor Joe. Doctor T told me "they never knew if I was going to hit them or swear at them when I woke up each time." Thank you very much that is just what I wanted to know.

I got back to my room at 8:00pm that evening. My daughter Kim was waiting in my room for me. I kept asking Kim to stay the night, another guilt trip.

The next morning I was up at 6:30am washed and dressed for Physical Therapy. I don't remember much about that day and slept through most of therapy but I was there. They said two of my golfing buddies came to therapy to see me, I don't remember.

My wound vac. had to be changed three times a week. Tina the nurse changed it every Monday, Wednesday and Friday. Doctor T scheduled his visits at the same time and along with him came his resident Doctor Joe, medical students and whoever else he dragged with him. Nurse Tina said she was going to put a tin cup out and start charging admission. The surgery was on Wednesday and on Sunday Doctor T did not come to see me and did not return until that Wednesday. When he walked into my room I said "you are not worried about me anymore because you missed three days and he said "you're right, I'm not worried," but he still continued to stop almost every day.

I showed my rear to every nurse and doctor in that hospital and anyone else who came into my room the day of the dressing change. Nurse Tina said she would have to start coming naked to do the change and I said only if you let me stuff your hole. There I go again. I meant only if she let me pack her wound if she had one. Of course every one thought this was funny, every one but me. Lord am I embarrassed.

The doctor and I even discussed surgery he was going to do on his relative and I told him to let his group do the surgery, but not himself. If by chance something bad happened he should not be the surgeon. I guess the relative has decided not to have the operation. I have never regretted having my back done. I am free of pain. To wake up at night and have no pain and walk down the hall even though I have to use the walker and drag the wound vac with me the operation has already changed my life. With the set back of the infection, I do not feel I went backwards far. I may have crabbed and bitched but I'm still plodding along. Surprised you, didn't I Doc. Patty told me what you said to her, "due to your mother's age you thought I would not put effort into getting better". I think you know now that I'm a very determined person. I hate people waiting on me. I rather do it my self. I think I'm my own worse enemy. I believe I can do everything and then I have to ask for help and that is what upsets me. I think I should be doing better.

I am still having a problem here in rehab when I have to go to the bathroom. When I say I have to go, I have to go right away or I mess myself. This is getting better I am not messing as much as I was. This has been quite and experience. I was never told this could happen.

Sometime should be spent on describing the food in rehab. It sucked, we even said we were going to protest one evening and toss our trays. Nurse Jo said she would put me in my room because I was the instigator of the revolt. We were just kidding around and the staff kidded along with us. You have to spice things up every now and then. But the food was nasty. George said I was just picky. So I told him he could eat my meals. By the time I drank that nasty Ensure that my lovely doctor ordered, I was not hungry for the food. George would take me to the cafeteria and I would get soup. They made real good soup. The food over there was much better. Everything tasted like peanut butter, I think that was due to the thrush I had in my mouth since January. That is nasty stuff and the blisters were very sore. Swish and swallow every day for weeks.

I am in my third week of rehab. Things are going well. My lower legs and feet are being washed in the evening and my stockings are being rinsed out and hung to dry. Josh, the male nurse is my care giver most of the time on evenings. He is a very nice young man. He always tells me about his two boys.

My girls are still washing my hair at noon every other day but today I washed it myself at the sink, another step forward. I don't care if the staff takes credit in the chart for washing it. Just as long as I can get it washed at least every other day.

I still need help in the morning to get my pants and socks on and my rear wiped. I still have the stitches in so I need assistance with that area as I do not need any more problems.

I am no longer having problems with going to the bathroom. I guess things are improving but not fast enough for me. I said I make a bad patient. I should be going home soon as I am doing most everything my self. I still have numbness in my right leg and hip area and the screw is still tightening when I exercise or walk. Not pain just pressure. I hope this gets better as time goes on.

OT therapist Pam gave me different helping aids to make things easier for me. She gave me something to put my socks on with. I tossed that as soon as she gave it to me. Needless to say I could have used it once I went home. I can put my socks on myself if I lay my knee bent on the bed and switch to the other the same way. I was given a reacher which I never used in rehab but will use at home. I think. I was offered elastic laces but of course I refused them as I was going to be able to do this myself once I got home. I was fooled again. Pam gave me a long shoe horn that works well. Last but not lease the handy ass wiper. Lord I hate that thing. It is long metal object that is bent in the middle and you put toilet paper on it. This upsets me, there has to be something different to use. I am going to design something else to use if I have to use it the rest of my life.

The time is coming when I will be discharged. Not soon enough for me. My muscle spasms are almost gone and I only take meds a couple times a day and when they change the wound vac.

I can now walk from my room to Physical Therapy and back to my room with my walker. When I first got here I could hardly walk across the room. And I'm doing most of my personal care myself. Except for the couple things I mentioned.

My concentration is much better. I can read the paper now and work the cross word puzzle. There is nothing more scary then thinking you are doing everything just fine and then have your kids tell you that you are still acting weird. Last names are hard to remember. I still have a problem once and a while. I always prided myself in remembering exact details.

CHAPTER 7

Roommates

Three weeks into my stay in rehab I got a room mate. She was just a teenager about nineteen years old. She refused all treatment and stayed up all night with her television on and getting calls at 3:00 am. Plus she wanted her boyfriend to stay all night. The nurse said, "It's up to your roommate as you share a room". I said, "Absolutely not. My husband does not stay". Me in my night shirt and no covers as it was so warm in the room and this young kid sitting there all night. The tip of the iceberg was when she was using ethnic slurs about certain nationalities and that was two of my grand children nationalities. I put a stop to that.

Her second day she asked to go outside so she can have a cigarette and they said she can go outside with a staff member but no smoking. She checked her self out AMA the next day.

My second roommate was a fifty two year old woman who had back surgery. We hit it off right from the first day. Bobby Jo and myself found out we lived in the same area. Perhaps we will see each other when we are shopping or out and about. We even liked the same room temperature. Bobby Jo was awake a lot at night, so we fit right in.

Bobby was having a bad time with her pain. The day before my discharge the new resident on rehab came to our room early in the morning and asked me how I was doing. I said, "fine I am going home tomorrow". His words were "you can not leave you are on to much pain meds". I said "right room, wrong patient". About two hours later he came and found me in Physical Therapy and apologized. No need to, it was an honest mistake. By this time I was only taking pills like twice a day.

I felt bad because the day I finally was discharged I never got to say good-by to Bobby Jo, she was in Physical Therapy.

CHAPTER 8

Discharge planning

The time has come to plan my discharge. What a fiasco! Every thing that could go wrong, went wrong. By the end of the week I was so frustrated and I wanted to strike out and hit some one. I know the Doctor kept telling me not to get depressed because I would cry. That was due to anger not depression.

My case worker, Anne, listened to someone else and received all the wrong information. Nothing was followed through on. First I was told that my Medicare and Blue Cross/Blue shield would not pay for my pic line at home or for my antibiotic and I would have to pay $ 102 a day. Then I was told that my insurance would not pay for my Wound Vac and supplies and we would have to pay $5,000 a month for the vac. By Friday my two Daughters that work at upstate, Debbie and Patty, asked for a family conference with my case worker Anne. Patty said, call KCI, the company that supplies the wound vac and put us on speaker phone". The call was made and they found out the caseworker never followed through and sent KCI the application for a wound vac. Twenty four to forty eight hours they would have known that my insurance did pay. After going home we found out that the insurance would have paid for the pic line, which the doctors got together and removed so I could go home. I was then put on cepral, oral meds. My girls were so mad because by this time I had stayed a week longer than I should have.

The hospital said I had to pay one thousand dollars for the week for staying longer then I should have. Doctor Way said absolute not. So far I have not received a bill for the extra week.

I can't even describe how upset I was through all this. I had no control over anything that was going on and that is something that I need to do, have control.

Arrangement had been made for me to go to Loreto Nursing and they would do the wound vac. They came and read my chart and found I did not qualify for that level of care. Thank god I did not have to go and be with the blue hair old ladies. Doctor T said "I am not going to be forced into a treatment that I feel is not safe for you". A wet to dry dressing was one of the options but was not acceptable.

By this time I was so upset and all I did was cry, swear and yell at everyone and usually it was to my family and Doctor T. I think back "was I a bitch?". I just wanted to go home.

Once the problems were sorted out and the forms completed everything fell into place. I think my girls were noted as trouble makers. But they got things done.

The wound vac was ordered and I was going home Tuesday. A walker with wheels was ordered for me. In—home nursing service and Physical Therapy, they were to come three times a week to my house. It seems impossible that everything is set. Let's cross our fingers.

Before my discharge my case worker came to my room and apologized for all the mistakes. I told her all I wanted to do is go home. She said, "I will take full responsibility and if your daughters want to follow up and do something it was alright with her". I don't care what they do, I just want out of here and the next time things will hopefully be different for other clients. The case worker said she knows now to follow through and not listen to someone else.

CHAPTER 9

The Big Day
March 5, 2008

5:30 am out of bed as usual. Help to bring my things into the bath room. Washed and dressed and out to breakfast with Ms. Dawn in the Recreational Room. I'm going to miss Peter and Dawn. They were a big part of my recovery. Thanks guys. Said my good bys to the patient I got to know.

Doctor T came to say good bye. I'm going to miss him. Little did I know that I was going to see a lot more of him in the near future?

My bags were packed with some help from the staff. My wound vac was delivered to the floor and the nurse had to put it on me. George arrived and the nurses are working on my wound. 11:00 am, I am ready to get out of here. Two of the nurses helped me out to the garage and a little shove with some helping hands and I was in the Durango and homeward bound. Thank the lord and anyone else who made it possible.

When we got home it was hard for me to believe that this day had finely come. Nothing had changed in the two months I was gone. Just that the weather is much nicer then when I went into the hospital in January. I can't wait to sleep in my own bed even though we had to switch sides due to the outlet for the wound vac.

Saint Joseph Nursing Service will be out tomorrow for an interview and inspection. I will have nurses to change the wound vac Monday, Wednesday and Friday. Physical Therapy was on Tuesday, Thursday and Friday. The home aide came on Tuesday and Thursday. I still think I don't need any help except for the wound care. Wrong again.

I am so weak from just riding home. Doctor T said I would tire easily but this is ridicules. I'm tired all the time. I even get tired just going to the bathroom. George has to wipe my butt because I still have my stitches that go from my bra line to inside my butt crack, plus the wound vac. But I have no pain.

Sorry doc that I keep saying this but I don't have any pain.

Chapter 10

Home Care
March 6th

Nurse Betty the overseer of my case arrived from the agency Wednesday 10:00am. The meeting went well and someone will come tomorrow, Thursday March 7th to change the dressing and pack the wound. Nurse Chuck became my wound changer. He is very nice and is very good at wound dressings. He will be my nurse until his own surgery on April 8th. Nurse Anne will take his place. I've gotten pretty good at detecting leaks in the barrier and my daughter Kim helps me if it leaks at night so I don't have to get the agency out here late night. Kim lives next door to me.

Aide Brenda comes at 3:00 pm on Tuesday and Thursday. I wish they would come early mornings before I have to go to the doctors so I'm clean. Kim and George assist me with washing and dressing myself doing the areas I can't reach on the days the aide is not here. Again they are helping me get my pants and socks on. I will master these things myself in time. I guess I have to expect that butt wiping will need to be done with that handy tool if I'm going to do it myself.

Doctor T said I may never be able to wipe my butt because of my short arms. He has one other male patient that has the same problem. I need some other type of tool then what they gave me to use if I have to use this until the day I die. This is not going to work for me. Maybe I can design something. A nurse friend of mine and myself are trying to come up with some ideas.

George went to the VFW to get me a wheel chair to get me to and from our family doctor. If he thinks I'm going to use that very long he's got another thought coming. My appointment is one week away and he says I have to use the chair.

March 15th, my appointment is today with my family physician Doctor Dennis. This will be the last time I use the chair. The walker is bad enough. I told George to just drop it off on our way home. The thought was good but I don't need to use it besides I need to walk for the exercise. Everyone is looking at me and my stupid machine is ringing and won't stop. I have to call the nursing service when I get home. Everything went well. Doctor Dennis was very interested in the operative site. I think everyone and their brother have seen my back. What's one more person? Upon arriving home I called the agency and a nurse came right away and took care of my wound and the machine. It is usually a simple matter.

I have been home two weeks now. I am still confined to the house. I call it house arrest. One of these days I am going over the wall.

When I go to see Doctor T on the 29th of March I will use a cane to get in his office and leave the walker in the car. Therapist Jane has tried me on the cane. The muscles in my legs and hips are still too weak. When I'm home alone I try the cane. Some times it's good, other times I stumble around. No more falls since the one in the hospital. Some close calls when I try more things independently. The therapist Jane laughs because if she tells me ten reps I do twelve. If she says twelve I do fifteen. I always want to get a few more if I can.

I still have a feeling in my right hip that a muscle is being tightened beyond its maximum. I don't know what it is. I joke and say I think the doctor put a self adjusting screw in. The more I do the tighter it gets. It is so frustrating.

I received a bill today for my stay in ICU from the hospital. I guess they forgot to send it to my insurance. It said 211,000 for one week in ICU payable in thirty days. Right on, I'll go to my grave owing it. I called the hospital and said "Send it to the insurance company".

My therapy is progressing but to me it seems very slow. I want everything better all at once.

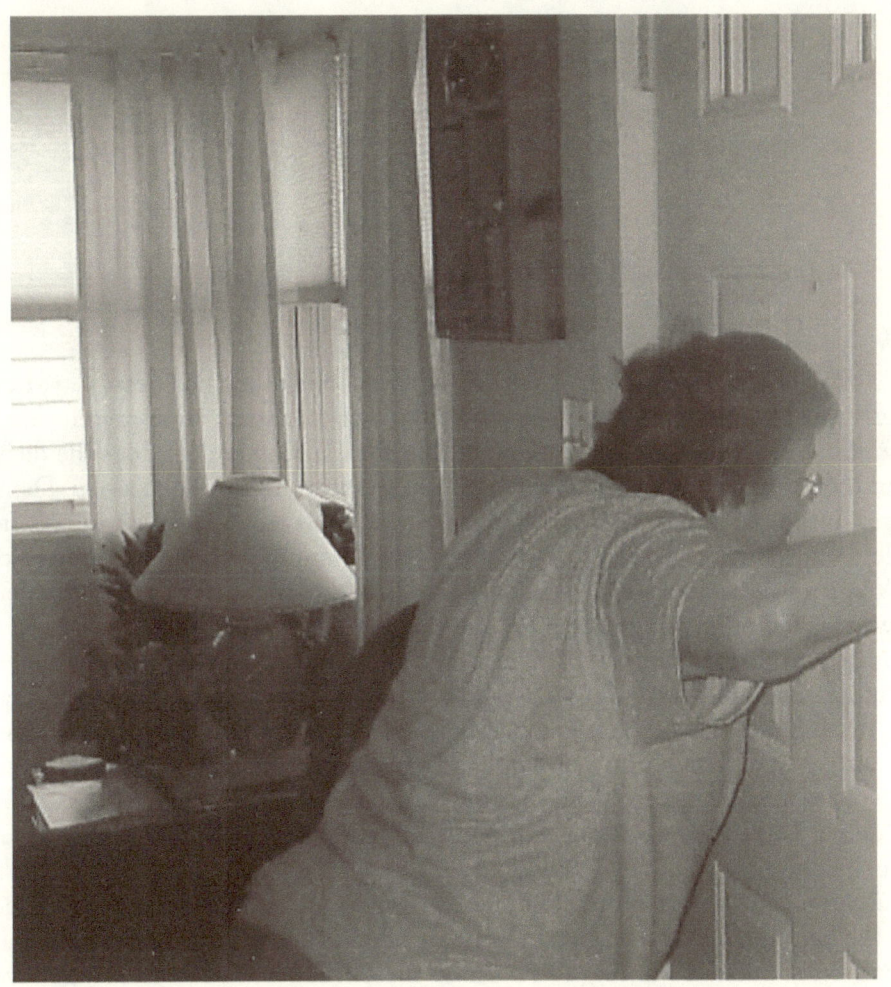

Pat doing push ups on the door.

Chapter 11

Home Adjustment

I have been doing more things for my self. I make the bed every day; I can wash most of myself except the hard areas. I still can not wipe myself due to the stitches. I help George get supper. I do the cooking and he does the dishes and then I take another nap. I do just so much then need to take a nap. Damn, I get so tired and then I get frustrated and I cry. I have read books and watched television so much that I've got to a point that I want to put my foot through the TV and burn the books in the middle of the living room. I make a terrible patient. I want to do everything now. The one thing I like is how the laundry is being done. George does a right fine job. The washer and dryer are in the basement. Physical Therapist Jane said she would teach me to go down the stairs and I said no that's fine. George is doing a good job. My Physical Therapist has me doing a number of exercises using rubber bands and leg and hand weights. When she leaves I take another nap. Then the aide comes and then another nap. I'm napped to death. I take pain meds one half hour before they come to change the vac and the dressing. It's not as bad as when they first started changing the wound. The muscles spasms are becoming less and less. I walk up and down from the kitchen to the bedrooms four times and then nap again. I know I complain a lot about not getting out and wanting to do things myself. I'm just a bitch. George says I must be feeling better. I would love to have a good argument but he never argues he would go out side first. He's always been like that. It frustrates me.

Picking up things from the floor is another chore. I do have a Grabber. I use that at times but try every now and then to reach out and pick up things. I can't reach straight down and probably never will be able to go straight down. I hate having people pick up things for me. I tell them I can do it my self.

Jane my Physical Therapist knows how frustrated I get and I want to do more things. I am so unsteady and off balance. She has me do a lot of balancing. She has also started taking me outside and I walk in the street. All I can do is to the next driveway and back and then time for a nap.

I will be going to Doctor T's office on Monday so the nurse will not be coming here that day. Insurance will not pay for a doctor's visit and the agency visit the same day. They are fixing a baggie with the dressing and wound vac barrier to take to him. I also am bringing him a box of Girl Scout Cookies. He made me drink that awful Ensure but I will be nice and take him something special for his patience and understanding.

CHAPTER 12

Removal of Sutures
March 29, 2008

The big day has arrived I'm finely getting to go somewhere even if it is only to the doctors. When I was called in the office I was using the cane and I gave him the cookies and he said "they are my favorites." Then I gave him the stuff for the dressing and he called Doctor Joe his resident down from the hospital to do the dressing and take the stitches out of my back. Doctor T is very happy with my progress, but of course I was complaining that I did not think I was progressing fast enough. Doctor T said he knows I'm ahead of my self.

Doctor T said he may be calling me to speak to some of his patients and I'm to tell them the bad and the good. I know I wanted to be able to speak to some one before I had surgery but they were not doing that at that time. I would be glad to do that if called. I have never regretted having the surgery I still do not have pain and I am no longer sleeping in the chair and I can walk without pain. I just have the problems with my hips. Mostly the right hip the screw tightening.

I have something new to wear four hours a day. As soon as I got here a rep. set me up with a bone stimulator. Dr. T said a young person bones start growing as soon as he cuts on them, but as you get older your bones lay down in the afternoon and takes a nap. I think he knew better than to tell me when you are old. I would have given him a knuckle sandwitch.

The doctor said I will probably wear it for nine months. I know him by now and I'm sure it will be at least nine months. He is always saying maybe. Doc you have to be assertive even if you think the patient will be upset. Afraid you might rile some ones feathers. I am only kidding.

I asked about a shower, but the boss said no, and I always do what he says. He said and "sometimes more, like your little walk at night". Let's just forget that one. I guess I have to think back what I was like in the hospital and I know I'm getting better. I believe you doc. I told George before we go home I want to go to lunch. I don't know when I will get out of the house again. I have my next appointment in three weeks. But things change quickly. We continue with the same routine every day. My therapist Jane takes me in the back yard and lets me hit golf balls. Doctor T said he never knew a therapist that shagged someone's golf balls for them. I think she knew that I enjoyed golfing. So she did it for me. Thanks Jane. I was bored with the inside exercise and I have a difficult time on the uneven ground and to bend over to pick up the balls is next to impossible. Sunday April 2nd I went to Mass at 7:30am. I escaped from the house for an hour and stopped after mass for breakfast. Monday my Therapist took me for a longer walk. I've been practicing with family members walking on the street and I can do ¼ of a mile.

CHAPTER 13

The Big Surprise
April 9, 2008

Woke up in the morning, got myself washed and dressed and kept feeling something picking under the barrier of the wound vac. Nurse Anne will be here around 9:00am. Got breakfast and made the bed. Boy is that ever picking and burning. The problem is on the right side of the back away from the incision line.

9:30 am Nurse Anne arrived and she proceeded to remove the dressing and barrier. When the barrier was removed she said something is wrong, you have a swollen area the size of a silver dollar under the skin. I had better phone the doctors office. Doctor T was in surgery but nurse Cat wanted me to come into the office so she can see it. This was Wednesday morning; George took me right down to their office. Nurse Cat drew a circle around it and said I had to return that afternoon for Doctor T to see my back. By the time I came back that afternoon it was the size of an orange under the skin. Doctor T went and got Doctor Larry to look at it. He is the plastic surgeon who seen me in the hospital. He said it had to be opened. I was given a choice to let Doctor T do it in his office or go and sit twelve hours in the ER at the hospital and then he would have to take me to the OR and open my whole back up. I told him to open it in the office. I did not know they had nothing to give me except the spray can of Lidocaine. I would say this was the worst since this all begin. He spoke to the infection doctor while he was opening it and squeezing everything out. Samples were sent to the lab. Doctor T said it may be MRSA. I think he knew it was that already because of the scaling. I am to return to his office tomorrow. I'll tell you doc if I had a pack of cigarettes when we left your office I would have smoked them all in five minutes.

April 10th we returned to Doctor T's office. The samples from the lab came back and confirmed I have MRSA. At this point I was put on 3200mg of antibiotics (Bactrian) after conference with the infection doctor from the hospital. I thought Doctor T was just going to look at the incision he made, wrong again it had to be drained again and re packed. I had been told to take two pain pills before I left home incase he had to drain it again. He knew damn well that was just what he was going to do. I think Nurse Cat felt sorry for me. It was not too bad. Just some foot shaking. I have to be on the antibiotics up to six weeks. **Back to his office on Friday and again same old thing.**

Make an appointment for tuesday and take two pain pills before you come here in case it has to be drained. You know damn well it will be squeezed. George says that the doctor packs a 4x4 in the opening. Nursing service was informed they had to change the dressing on Saturday and Sunday.

I think the sulfur is making me sick to my stomach and gives me diarrhea and hives I'm getting a reaction to the sulfur. April 13th back to the doctor's office. I'm starting to hate this place. More stuff being squeezed out.

When I told the doctor I was walking a ¼ of a mile he told me to go a half a mile. If it hurts stop but if you are just tired then suck it up and go some more. I told him he was Simon Lagree. (Slave driver's boss) I feel more tired and seem to rest more often. I think it has something to do with the infection.

April 14th. Back to his office I was told not to come back for one week. He asked me how I was feeling as I was looking good and I said out side of feeling pregnant from the nausea from taking the sulfur, having the shits and scratching my brains out. I guess I'm fine. Nurse Cat gave me a script for benadryl for the itch. Nursing service is to come every day and re-pack the wound.

April 21st my next appointment with the doctor. I am feeling real fine and should be getting off house arrest. I am still unable to take a shower because of the open wound. The day is getting closer I'm going to get in the shower for two hours. I do not have to see Doctor T for two weeks. I asked doctor T if I could put the bone stimulator on my arms and make them grow one or two inches so I could reach my behind so I don't have to use that tool to wipe.

CHAPTER 14

Back to Rehab

May 10th check up with Doctor Way. Everyone has to go back to rehab for a follow up. Today is my day.

I drove myself to the hospital after I had to have my granddaughter Kristy tie my shoe laces. Lord I hated asking her to do this. I will ask at rehab for a pair of elastic laces. They wanted to give me them when I was there as a patient and I was determined not to use them. I refused to admit that I needed them I was going to be able to do my shoes myself. This is real hard to say, I can't. Like I said I'm my own worse enemy. I feel like I could bungee jump or sky dive or anything else I want to do. My head says yes and my body says no.

My goal at this point is to walk outside without my cane and not be afraid I will fall. I also want to start my golf leagues, which is not happening at this point.

My check up went well. Doctor Way could not understand why I'm not in out side Physical Therapy until I told her that I had been on house arrest with MRCA. Until the wound closed no therapy place would take me. I start outside Therapy on June 2nd.

I ran into the supervisor who heads rehab floor. I asked her about my room mate but she said she does not remember her. She only remembers the ones that caused trouble. I guess that was me. Oh well, we got things happening. May 29th saw Doctor T for a scheduled appointment. Still have problem with right hip the more I exercise the more it feels like it is tightening on me. Nurse Cat gave me a shot in my hip. They think it may be my bursa that it is inflamed. Things are going well. We don't want to brag too much. My wound has closed up.

I brought doc another box of Girl Scout cookies, Samoas. He said these are his favorite. "A lot nicer than a can of Ensure Doc"—I'm thinking. I'm still waiting for our drink together.

Chapter 15

May 31, 2008
Shower Day

The big day has finely come to the Martin's house. My back is healed and the scabs are gone. "I CAN TAKE A SHOWER". It has been four months. I'm not sure if I know what to do. This feels great.

George is doing a funeral with the rifle squad from the Legion. I arrived at the post to wait for him and I told who was there I finely took a shower and no one has to stand down wind from me any more. Give me a B/V and ginger this from a diet pepsi drinker.

About this time the guys got back and the Deacon, Jay and I got celebrating my big feat for the day. Me, who always drinks diet soda, ended up having five mixed drinks. I was a happy camper that day. Do you know what it's like to take a shower after four months? I guess this was not normal for me but I was in the best spirits I've been in since long before the surgery. Now if I did not have to use that handy ass wiper. There has to be a better way to handle this problem. We are working on it.

By this time I have gone for a hair cut and new glasses. I am starting to feel like a human being again. We take things for granted so often. I can walk in a store without using a cart to lean on. George will say, "do you want a cart?". No, just my cane and I am walking straight. It is hard to believe.

I have been talking about volunteering in rehab. I feel like giving something back for everything they did for me. I would be playing cards, games or reading or just sitting with the patients. So many clients do not have anyone to visit with them. So I set up an appointment and spoke to the volunteer office and had my interview and went to the health office to be cleared. I got my picture taken for my ID. Now it's just getting my orientation in and picking a day that is convent for every one.

I was told if I get an open cut or sore I have to stay away because of the MRSA

I am still unable to do some things. Like marching in the Memorial Day parades. So the Post has me taking pictures. Had these two taken just to bust your chops Doctor T. You can tell I am doing better. Wanted to see what your reaction would be. Love to see your face get red.

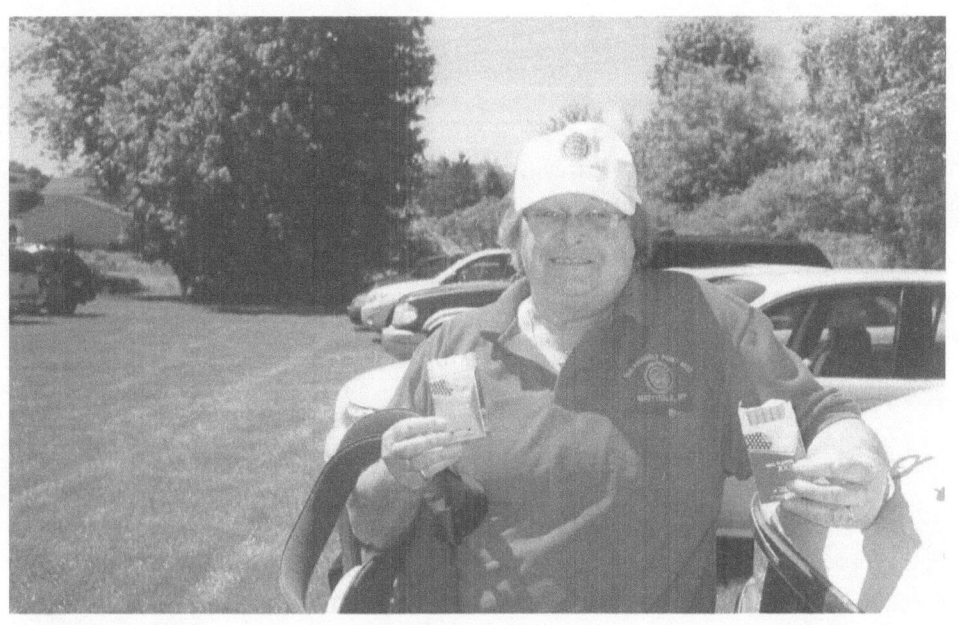

Pat with open cigarettes.

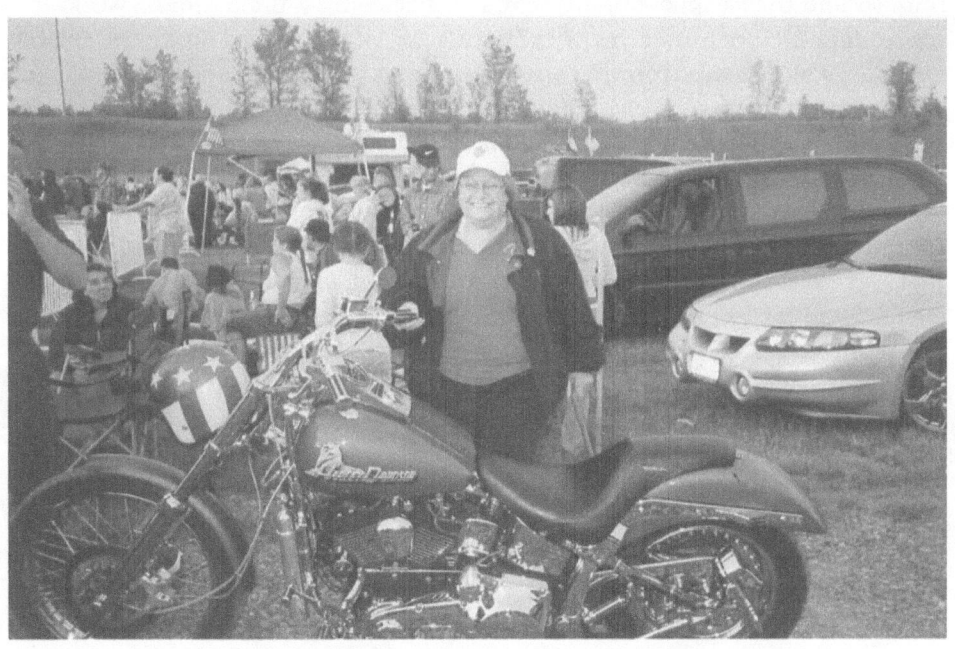

Picture two not my bike. Wanted you to think I was riding this.

CHAPTER 16

Physical Therapy
Monday June 2, 2008

The day has come when I get to exercise with other people. I met with my Therapist Doctor Smart. He set me up with a program to strengthen my back muscles and the weakness in my hips. I will be coming three times a week. It is really funny Doctor Smart was just a "wanna-be" be when I had my knees replaced ten years ago. He was worrying about his exams coming up and was still living with his parents. As soon as I walked in I remembered him. He has not changed. He is now married has two children and has his own work place.

I am working with rubber bands for my back muscles and ten lbs of weights but only to my shoulders. The stepping stool bothers my hip a lot. Hamstring stretches. Rear kicks, five lbs. Side leg lifts are very hard for me to do. I can do them without weight. I am unable to do the right leg even with only one lb. weight. I do the cross-trainer for ten minutes on level four and the tread mill at one point seven.

The staff is real nice and helpful and glad to be of help to the clients. I am in my third week of therapy and have increased every thing. My hip is still bothering me. But this has been a problem since right after the surgery. It feels like something tightening. The therapist advised me to call the doctors office and inform them that the injection Nurse Cat gave three weeks ago did not help. So I did, and Cat said I should cut back on therapy so now they are only letting me do the arms workout. No leg exercise. I can work through the screw tightening because it's not pain just discomfort with pressure, but they say no.

I am now back in Aquatics. It feels wonderful, the warm water, but I still have the pressure in the right hip and the numbness from the edge of my butt to the side of my knee. I feel it is a muscle and that is why I have to walk with a cane when outdoors, as I am off balance. Inside I can walk without my cane but still somewhat unsteady. Stairs are the worst. I have to pull myself up each step using my right hand and it really bothers my right hip. I hate to complain because I am so much better than before the surgery. I have not taken pain pills since I had the staff infection. It is now Saturday, June 27, 2008. I have had two sessions of water therapy and my hip still feels the same. I was there on Thursday and again on Friday. Debbie, the assistant, has had me both times.

I almost got in a fight with some eighty year old lady in the locker room. I was struggling to put my socks on, which I can do myself it just takes me some time. She grabbed the sock and put it on my foot and just as quick grabbed the other one and put that one on also before I could say no thank you I can do it myself. This up set me because if I needed help I would have asked or gone home without putting them on. Maybe I'm to pig headed but I want to do it myself.

I have made up names for the staff at therapy and Aquatics. Jim, the complainer, but a very good worker, Adonis, the muscle bound and the young one, The Learner. They all seem to be very concernrd about your well being. The serious one (I will let you think about who that is.) is always right there questioning you on everything and making suggestions.

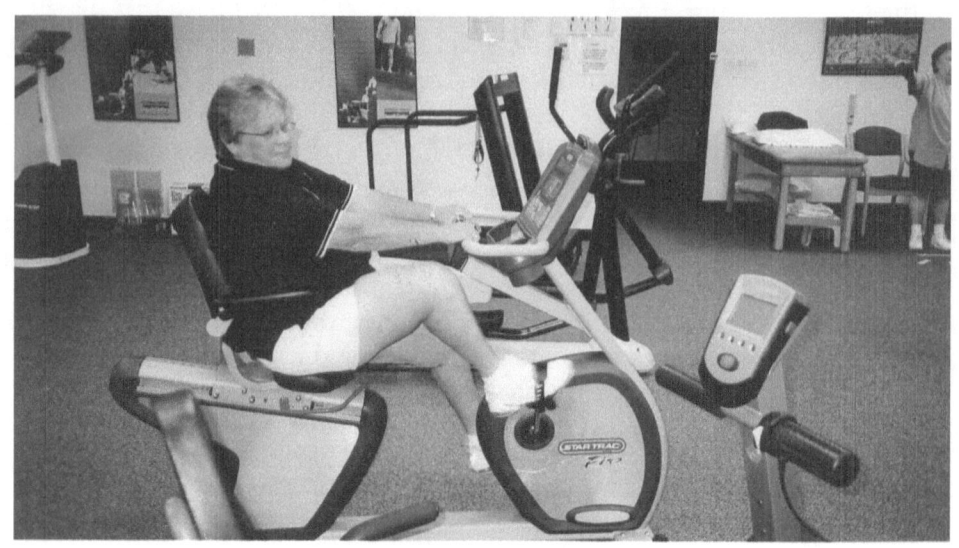

Pat (on bike at therapy)

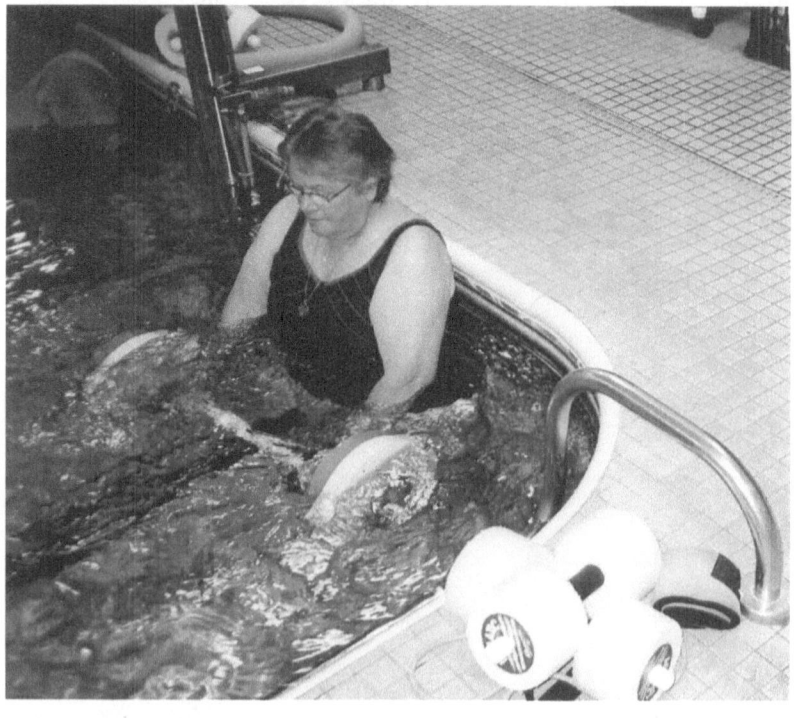

Pat (In the pool doing water the therapy)

CHAPTER 17

The Impossible

Every week I find something I can't conquer. June 14th installation dinner. George is Commander again for the American Legion Post and our son George jr. is the Sons Commander and I was elected president of the Auxiliary. I went out bought a new skirt, blouse, shoes and pantyhose. This was my first big outing since my surgery. Well, let me tell you, after trying for ten minutes to get those damn pantyhose on, I finally had to ask George to put my right foot in them. He said "you better call Kim next door and have her do them". I said "absolutely not". She had to put my pants on me in the hospital and she is not going to put my stockings on me. Have you ever seen a six foot, two hundred and sixty pound man put pantyhose on his wife? Let me tell you it is not a pretty site. We were both laughing so hard by the time we got done. It's a good thing I can laugh about some things. I will never wear panty hose in my lifetime again unless I can put them on myself. Also, I could not conquer the shoes. They were only slip on with very little support. I was staggering all over the place. I took my sneakers with us and put them on whenever I had to do any walking. My balance is still not right I stagger around if I walk without a cane. I'm starting to hate that also. Bitch, bitch, bitch never satisfied.

The day I messed my clothes before I got home from the store because I did not have my trusty ass wiper on me. I was crying and screaming and throwing things in the bathroom. If I could have got my hands at that moment on the short heavy Italian, Doc I would have killed you. I walked out of the john bare ass and my daughter Kim was standing in the living room and said, "What the hell are you doing?" She got me laughing describing to me how I sounded when I was ranting and raving. I got caught with my pants down again. I just get so upset not being able to wipe myself. The latest incident was Saturday June 21st. I got up at 6:00am and was not feeling well. I realized I was going to be sick. Guess what I can't bend over the toilet and vomit. I had to kneel on the floor and do it. George said "Why didn't you use the sink or trash can." At a moment like this you are just trying to not make a mess. I was not thinking of anything else.

I am now golfing in one of my four leagues. It is a struggle to put the tee in the ground and nine times out of ten the ball falls off the tee on the first attempt. I have to reach out not down to put it in the ground. If I have my rain suit on then I have to get someone else to tee up for me as I do not have enough flexibility. I need a suction cup on the end of my putter so I can get the ball out of the hole. I can't tie my golf shoes so someone else does that. I have some real good friends that are fine with helping me or maybe they are just afraid what I might do if I get upset. Ha Ha. These things bother me. By the end of nine holes I'm ready to quit because of struggling with the tee. But I guess I should be happy that I'm getting out. My head tells me I can golf all my leagues but my body still says no. It's my right hip that keeps nagging at me.

My girl friend and I are still working on a different butt wiper. We haven't quite mastered it. I know the name will have to be something other then ass or butt wiper.

Also if I go to a restaurant we always sit in a booth. Not any more unless I am seated on the outside as it is too difficult to get across the seat to get out. Just everyday things you take for granted can turn out to be a chore. The worst thing anyone can do is say let me do it. At least for me it is difficult to accept help. If I need someone's help I will ask, ok?

I also know I can't pull weeds unless I sit down to do it. I was upset that my Roses were not weeded so I decided to do it myself. Instead of sitting on the rock garden wall I leaned against the sun room and reached out and weeded three beds. George said whom did you hurt, just yourself. O my god I had such muscles spasms for three days. I guess I showed everyone I could do it. Pig headed.

CHAPTER 18

Typhoid Annie

I had to have blood work done recently and my crit was low. I think it is because of the Thalasimia Minor but Doctor Dennis referred me to a doctor to have a colonoscopy and endoscopy. I also had to go and have an anemia panel done. I asked Doctor T if this was necessary. He said I'm a bone doctor not medical. Do what your family doctor says. Every doctor I go to I have to tell them I am a carrier of MRSA. So I will be the last patient of the day. The doctor who is doing the procedure is none other then doctor Mike whom I worked with in the procto room when I worked at the hospital.

"I thought you would be retired by now" and his reply was "every time I go home to tell my wife I am retiring she tells me she's pregnant". I am down for July 8th at 2:00 pm for the procedure and the last patient of the day.

I made an appointment to have a pap smear and guess what? The same thing, at the end of the day.

I never want this MRSA to flare back up and come back on me. But there is always the possibility. The doctors don't want to commit themselves. I know it was brought into my home by the agency as they were treating someone else in my area with MRSA and then came to my house for dressing changes. How do you prove this and if I could what good would it do. I would still be a carrier and it will still be in my body and will not go away. If I get a cut or have an opening I have to stay away from the population. That is why I say I am Typhoid Annie.

July 8th, this is the day for the colonoscopy and endoscopy. The prep was terrible having to use the special tool and my muscles are not fully back to normal. I have to stay near the crapper. I Arrived at the center at one pm, filled out all the papers, and was put into a private room. I told them this is the first and last time I come to this place. Never felt a thing. They sure gave me some good stuff. I still will not come back. That prep just blew my mind. Doctor Mike came in and said the bottom area was fine I had one polyp, but I was bleeding in my stomach. Now I will have to wait for my family doctor to call. The doctor thought it was from the anti-inflamatories so I was switched back to Arthotec. This appears to be working well.

CHAPTER 19

Pay Back Time.

We have been invited to my great nephew's graduation. It is at the War Memorial, downtown. I can't believe I had no pain after parking three blocks away, walking all the way there. I only had the problem with the right hip. I used a cane and it helps to balance me when I walk.

Today is pay back time Laurie. Remember the brace and the tassels. Well this is just for you. I took this brace out of the trash bag this morning Sunday the 30th of June. George put it away when he brought it home in February. All this time I thought the brace was a tan color. As you can see it is very white. I guess I was still nuts in rehab at least for a while.

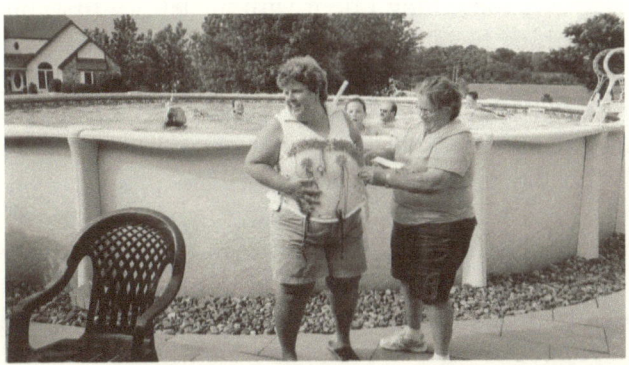

Laurie with my brace with added items just for her.

I look forward to these parties and up coming weddings without dread of being in pain and not wanting to attend.

CHAPTER 20

Only Time Will Tell

I can't believe how well I feel. This is the best in years. Dr. T said I can't make your back like it was when you were a teenager. It's been to many years since I was a teen for me to remember. But this is the best I've been in at least five years. (I HAVE NO PAIN). I have some problems with balance and weak hip muscles. I may not be able to master certain parts of my normal daily activities, like tying my shoes. Bending straight down, I have to lean out and down. With my artificial knees I am unable to squat. I am unable to turn and look behind myself unless I turn my whole body. I will never be able to wipe my rear without the trusty tool. I still have a problem with my right hip and I need my cane to walk any distance and to lift my leg over something I do it with my left leg first. But to be free of pain is beyond anything I can imagine.

July has been a roller coaster ride for me, I received a call from Therapy that I can no longer get Physical Therapy, Congress voted down extended therapy for extenuating circumstances. I can pay out of pocket or wait for congress to return after the holiday to re vote or take a wellness program that I have to pay for myself.

Everyone at therapy is calling Congressman Jim Walsh office in Syracuse. And find out what he can do to help us. I left a message for Marty who works in the Syracuse office of Congressman Walsh, he handles all Medicare issues. He will call me tomorrow or I am to phone him. July 3rd Marty from Walsh's office phoned, but I was at a meeting. So I phoned when I got home. I left him a message. I guess we are playing phone tag. I am sure it will be after the holiday tomorrow when I hear from him.

I hope something can be done about this matter. Elections are coming up in November and there are seniors out there who are having the same problems in regards to their health care. A large majority of the voting population are senior citizens. Congressman Jim Walsh office called back, Marty did not know what I was talking about. Someone from the Washington's office will call me. I was informed today that there was to be a re-vote this week.

It is now the second week of July and congress over rode the Presidents veto and passed the bill we have been waiting for. Thank you. I resume my Therapy Monday and my wellness program is on hold. My appointment on July 22nd with the doctor was not a good visit. I was upset with the way I walk without my cane. My hip was bothering me and I needed another shot. I was still having a couple problems that the doctor had to check out.

Doctor T was upset with me when I said I was trying to ride my bike outside. He said at sixty seven years old I should not be doing certain things and riding a bike was one of them. That really upset me because 67 is just a number. I told him if I felt good there is no reason why I can't do it. Taking long walks and having no hip pain, and swimming in the pool, taking care of my house, grocery shopping and doing outdoor activities like golfing is just a few things I want to be doing without having problems.

If he had said that I was not ready for bike riding and should start out on the stationary bike then I may have been agreeable, maybe not because I was quite upset over my bathroom problem. But don't say because of age.

I will apologize to him at my next visit on August 21st. I told my girlfriend this and she acted like she was going to faint. I'm not that stubborn am I. I thought I was a very easy going person.

CHAPTER 21

The Ride

This will be the last chapter in my story. I pray that I continue gaining ground and perhaps I have another ten years that I can enjoy life without pain is beyond anything I can imagine.

If I can be of help to someone else who has chronic pain and living a life that is less then good, I hope my story will be helpful in helping them make the big decision to have surgery or not.

I can recommend a doctor that is not only excellent in his field but also has compassion for his patients. If you have any doubts just call me and see how well I am doing.

I have been volunteering in rehab for the past three Tuesday's. It has opened my eyes to how lucky I am. I want to give back for all the help they did for me. I just have to look around and see the clients struggling to accomplish their every day chores it makes me think back to when I was in the same boat.

On May 22nd 2009 I will be 68 years old and I am doing a benefit for the children cancer unit at upstate. Thirty of us are going to ride bikes on the Erie Cannel 68 miles. Thirty 34 miles on the 22nd and 34 back on the 23rd and all donations will be going to the kids.

So Doctor T, do you think I can complete this ride. I believe I can with training all winter and therapy is also instructing me on different exercises. I have been riding a stationery bike every day and now I can at least get on my outside bike and not feel like I'm going to kill myself. I have to admit you were right again. I was not ready last month. I think you know it is very hard for me to say I was wrong and you are right. (OUCH). Enjoy the wine. That was my way of saying, you're right, again.

Doctor T you will have a special invitation when the ride is done to come to the dinner, so keep the afternoon of May 23, 2009 free. I would challenge you to the ride both the 22nd and 23rd but I know you are a very busy person, but it would have been fun to see who would quit first. It would not be me.

Don't forget the promise you made and the drink we are to have. Again I can never repay you for every thing you have done for me. Guess what? "I STILL DO NOT HAVE PAIN".

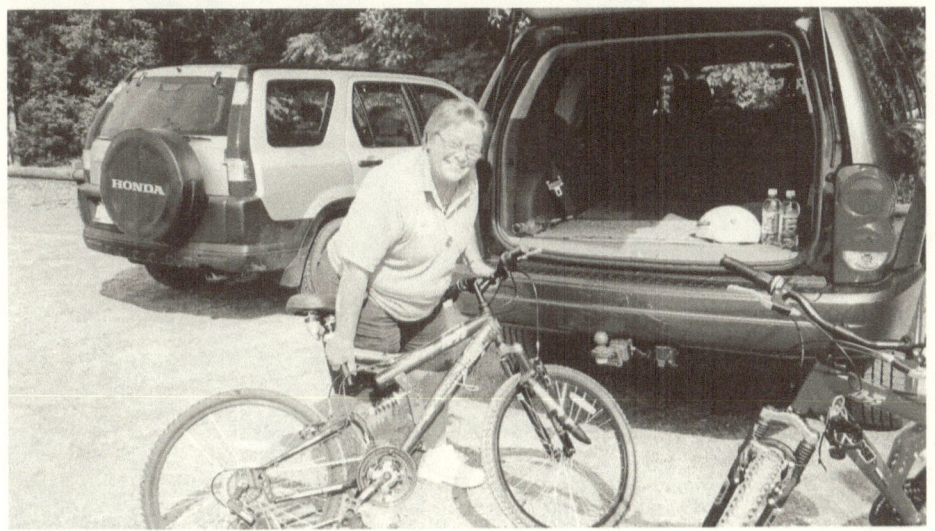

After a ride.

www.ingramcontent.com/pod-product-compliance
Lightning Source LLC
Chambersburg PA
CBHW031330290526
45784CB00014B/2487